THE GIRL FROM ORCHARD PARK WITH ALOPECIA

Based On A True Story

Delena Smith

Order this book online at www.trafford.com
or email orders@trafford.com

Most Trafford titles are also available at major online book retailers.

Printed in the United States of America.

ISBN: 978-1-4669-4340-7 (sc)
ISBN: 978-1-4669-4341-4 (hc)
ISBN: 978-1-4669-4339-1 (e)

Library of Congress Control Number: 2012910910

Trafford rev. 06/20/2012

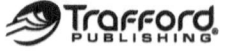 www.trafford.com

North America & international
toll-free: 1 888 232 4444 (USA & Canada)
phone: 250 383 6864 ♦ fax: 812 355 4082

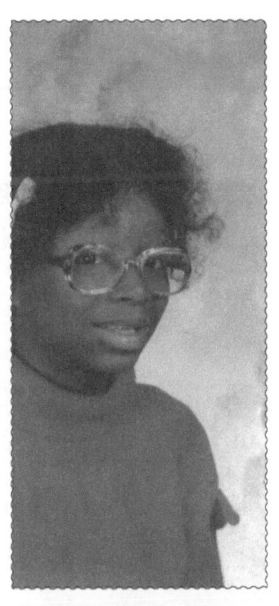
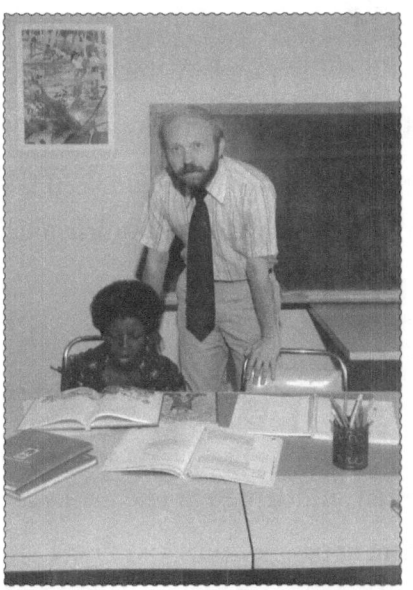
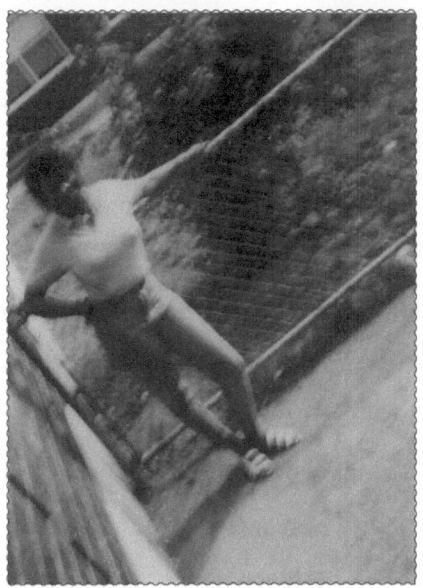
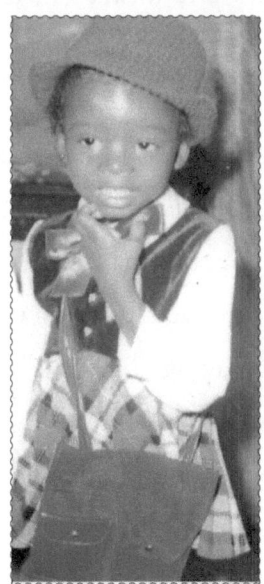

*A*s the summer of '77 began, my grandma and mom decided that my sister and I were going to go to my auntie chilly's in L.A. for a couple of weeks. The trip was fun but long, and everyone was happy when my sister and I returned home. But that's when all the problems started. And although I did not learn this fact until much later, I had developed the alopecia hair disease.

I was forced to learn from an early age that part of being

Special and different meant living in a big place with many diriment people and a lot of big buildings . . . and that sometimes that world wasn't a nice place to live.

We lived in the inner city section of Boston Massachusetts aka "the ghetto" but I attended the Harvard Kent elementary school, the Michael Angelo middle school, and Charlestown high school in the suburban part of the city in Charlestown. I also went to these schools on a special bus. I can still hear my grandma now saying "here it is" as we heard the 'beep beep" of that little bus in front of the house. I remember the taunting calls from the neighborhood children saying "why is she on the small bus" and saying to myself . . . . here we go again with a day full of questions.

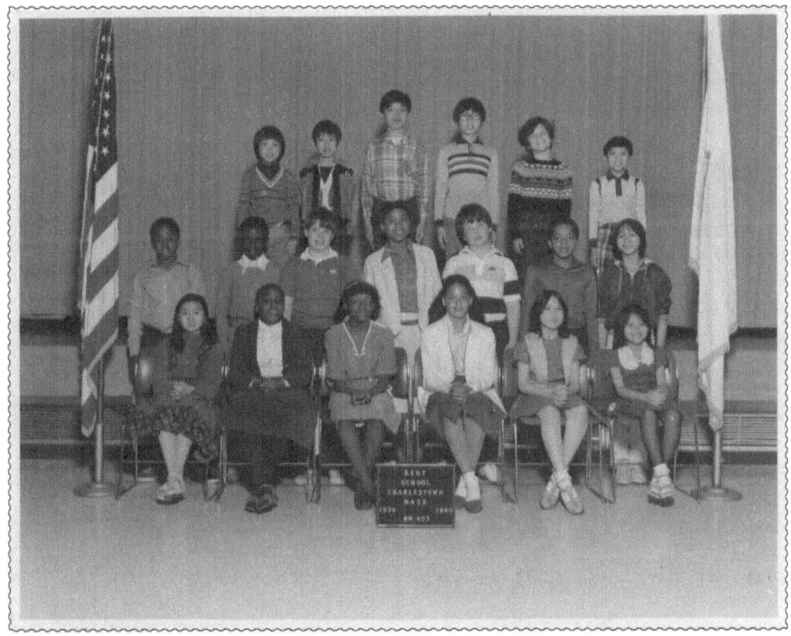

kids would do all types of things to me like pick fights with me, call me names, laugh at me like I was a clown all the time and do mean things to me as a little girl, all the time. They all made fun of me. They all thought that I was a joke. I was mentally messed up and they had no idea of the nice caring & loving person I truly was. Sometimes I would feel that I wasn't wanted but I would always try to fit in anyway. And although I had a few girlfriends, most of them wouldn't play with me. They didn't want to be around me because I wasn't "like them". I was going bald and didn't know why. And when I was feeling extremely depressed my grandma would say to me "lets go to our special store girl, Dee's wig salon."

When we got there

My grandma would gently ask, "What do you want?" my timid answer always being "I don't know grandma."

One Saturday

After hanging out with my grandma, I went to the "corner" store called "brown's" wearing my new wig. As I was heading home, I got that sickening feeling in the pit of my stomach . . . . something's not right. I can hear them behind me . . . . girls . . . walking, talking . . . . doing their best to taunt me. Saying things like . . . .

"is that her hair?" and

"I don't think so girl" . . . and

"Why she wear those wigs"

"I don't know maybe she sick or something"

They took my wig and threw it in the sewer, forcing me to go home without my safety net. and as they snickered and laughed, I just kept walking, saying to myself, "I wish I could go some place where people don't notice my hair." here are a bunch of unanswered questions, then my sister and brother, why me? I hated the way that I looked, wishing I could just take it off and give it away thinking to myself, the main question was where was where exactly did it come from? And why was I picked to have it good? The main problem I had was why wasn't I educated about it more? Just thinking about the days when I was going to summer camp I could never be like the other girls just getting in the water why was I the one who always had to wear swimming caps? Here are more questions! And never mind taking a shower in the cabin. Embarrassed! Girls would have their ponytails and I couldn't do it, more questions to ask. Going to high school on public transportation, in front of my house, I couldn't skip school grandma and grandpa, also known as Paul. They would see me as I would be getting on the bus to make sure I did so safely. Kids would tease me still though. On the school bus I would sit in the back, hoping I wouldn't be noticed. Thinking they would forget about me today and wouldn't tease me today. By then, here we go again with the teasing. As I was young, knowing when I was little, I looked like a pencil, very skinny and some people would call me "girl Mrs. basely". With my glasses on I never could have the boys. They acted like they were my boyfriends one minute, but really throughout time, they thought I was an ugly girl; it would really cause me to be even more insecure than I was. I never wanted to be around a lot of people when I was younger. I had a very hard time dealing with learning. It was very difficult to do, having alopecia and not knowing what I had until I got older. I wanted to understand more about myself and the disease, and what it would be like being pregnant. Walking around in school with the crowded kids always yelling, the ones whispering something about me were always easy to spot, but I would rarely lift my head up. I would just clutch onto my school books and fix my prescribed eyeglasses, walking quickly to my next class in embarrassment. I heard them always laughing in the background & the tones of their chuckles are still so fresh in my mind "ha haha". I became depressed and started to have angry feelings of feeling I was stupid and feeling like I was dumb or crazy. I felt like that about myself for most of the earlier part of my life, for a long time it happened to me. From grammar school, to high school and then some. Girls would just want to fight me for no real reason, just so they could see what's under my hair/wig. Knowing what I know now I see that my grandmother & mom spent a lot of time at the doctor's office with me, where I had to go in so that they could use me as a guinea pig pretty much. Injecting my head with needles, I also had extensive radiation done on me. Not long after so much being done, I begged my mom & grandma "please don't send me back there so they can't do that anymore to me. I hate it there!" saying to family members that I didn't want to go back again, I didn't want to be in pain anymore. It hurt my head and it stayed in pain. Please lord help! So my grandma finally stopped taking me back there anymore, her and mom spent money, buying wigs for me. Growing up that was my "safety net" to me, my hair, and my wigs. Having the type of family that I had been warm and loving when it came down to my special problem, being different than everybody in my family. Thinking god made nobody perfect, but we all need to give people respect. It was very difficult for me to be with a lot of children in the class, I was scared and it was hard to learn & focus. I couldn't think around people and didn't like crowds. I tried to keep them small if I could because at that time I had real bad nerves and couldn't learn the way I should or could. only my faith in the lord made me not want to kill myself, I can just thank the lord for keeping me here, a stronger person some of my friends I knew just didn't like me, but my sister, she was the rock of the family. Any time there was a problem with me she was always there. If not just her, many of my family members would help me. She always made me feel special in her own way. We have a very different and special love for each other, me and my sister! My grandma is the rose of the whole family, she is the one that makes the family complete. Her whole family grew strong, and "it" without her is a lost place to me. My grandma is the shining light of the family, my mom & grandma, without them in my life it would've been a lot of dark days for me. There are all kinds of dark secrets, this was the hard one. I had to tell the whole world, hoping people can feel what I felt. I can remember going with my father for the holidays, me and my sister in Albany, new York in the early 70's when I was between my early talking years, I was around 4. I remember my father cooking a pig, which took most of the day to cook it. He would be in the back yard of his apartment that he was renting at the time. For the rest of the days we spent together, and had the best holiday memories to cherish.

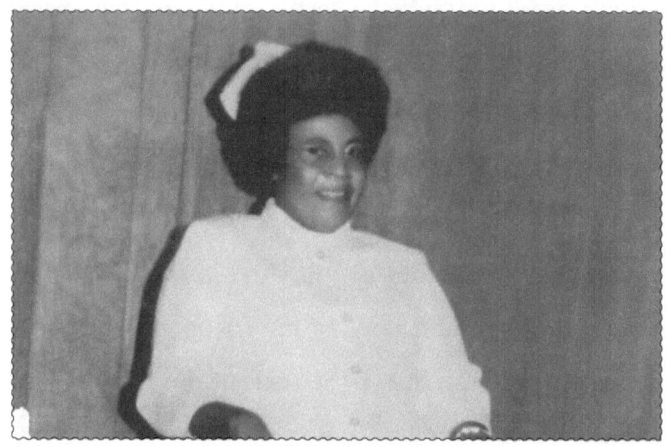

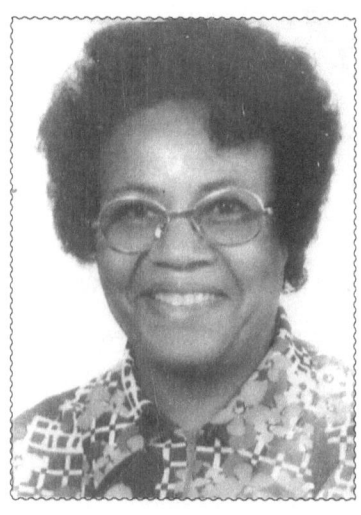

I remember my sister & I had some fun times with our dad, my grandmother on my dad's side lived in Albany as well. She always did stuff with me and my sister, whether it was going to church to pray, going fishing on a boat, or just on the creek. My grandma made it to be 102. She never drank or put drugs into her body. That good living and good health that she taught me had me growing up where there were all types of special people around. Coming from the "big break city" most people who were meant to had become famous already. Becoming one more shining star one day as I grew up never came to my mind. I came to have my teenage ways which some of them I wish I could take back but as we know, some things we just can't take back. The lord got me through it all though, I can't put my hands threw my hair like other girls. It seems like they would bother me because they knew I didn't have hair like them, they knew it was a wig. As a girl some things started looking different in my life to me, finally I can talk about things and some people can relate to it, with or without alopecia. It is a different disease to have to deal with being a little girl living in the projects. I know some kids with diseases have a lot of problems with them. Sometimes they become an inside problem to your mind and body. after being the ugly duckling for so long, now it was time to turn into a beautiful swan.

I was born in Albany New York on November 12, 1967 with my proud parents Janice & Gerald. As time went on we went back to the Massachusetts area, living in a city project nicknamed "o.p." for Orchard Park with my mother and grandma as a little girl having alopecia and not knowing what it was at the time, living in the orchard park project I saw most of being teased, bullied, picked on & name called. growing up after living with this disorder daily & learning that I was a special person that came from the urban neighborhood, as a lady I became a wife and mother of 4 children over time, that, I never thought I'd be around long enough to live to see it from my earlier days. today, I am focused on raising my other son and presently still living in Massachusetts with my family in good health. my brothers, sisters and other family members all are still very supportive to me & them. I can proudly say that I am a grandma myself to my 2 loving grand babies. I can never express in words just how happy to see these days in my life I am. there were a lot of fallen angels and painful days to remember that are in the past now but never forgotten in my mind. they are like old urban ghost stories to me in my dreams and soul to always be remembered. as I go back into my memory banks and throughout time there has been all kinds of bad times of me being tormented. maybe I was at the wrong place at the wrong time most of the time, but when I look at life after all the things I've lived through, I really turned out to be one of the lucky ones to still be alive to shed light on my generation's era. it was the late part of1978 & my mom had sent me to the store, it was just at the corner you could see it from my building.

this day the wind & snow was blowing so hard that you couldn't see down the street. I was the oldest so I had to be the one to go to the store alone and at this time it was one of the 1st times I had to act like I was the oldest, which I was. it was so cold that day, I remember walking & as I was halfway to the store, and a man stopped me and said "give me your money! not knowing all I had was what mom had given me to get bread and milk which wasn't much. I said to the man "I don't have money but don't kill me please". he had a gun and I started to cry but at the same time I was praying and I looked up and he was going to let me go although he had took my money but not my life, thank the lord. being a proud mother of my boys there were some things that I had to sit down and explain to my guys, like that their mother had a hair problem. at the time I dont really think they know what I was really talking about until they got older when they understood better later on in life. I come across as an educater of alopecia to them, regarding our history. as time went by I ended up meeting my 2 eldest boys' dad mr man. he was the man that could step up to the plate for me & be someone I can have to hold and talk to. most men were scared of what people said. he was the first guy that just didn't look at me like that. he saw something else in me that back then, I didn't see in myself. and that's how it went, one of the best things that happened in my life at that time. they said it would not last but with the man upstairs he was on my side so how could I go wrong? that's what I said after getting older, back then, I was thinking I knew where my alopecia came from. it was when I was younger more people needed to be educated about the hair / skin disorder. back then at that time, is when it counted the most. I can remember my uncle and aunt coming early in the morning just before I went off for school. what a gift that was to brighten my days. those were just some of the things that my family did to show me that they really love me and can feel some of what I feel. like when other children would take my wig off and throw it around like it was a towel. that stuck with me. and they thought it was funny at the time. taking the only thing I had for security to my life. I have had a lot of rough days to remember. even crazy days of thinking about doing the unthinkable to myself. that's why I have to dedicate my book to all of the people that have the alopecia hair disease. this problem and any other disorder that is difficult to live with but as we know, god didn't make anyone perfect in this world besides himself, never judge a book by its cover. and I do hope this book makes a change for others in this world. alopecia is not a disease you can die from, you just have it for a lifetime. that to me was the worse to find out. the skin or hair part of it isn't something I liked to hear about either. but now I understand that there are millions of people throughout the world dealing with the same issues I have been dealing with all these years. I'm confident that people will relate to me. it has become more familiar for me to see it, it's really out there in the world, I have seen children and other adults, born like me living life as they should be. it's important to be visible online because there are still lots of people that don't want anyone to know what they have. I just want people to know that you are not alone in this. we all live life and I know how it feels, don't be afraid. speak up and you will be heard that is the American way, I think of all the days when my grandma would stand up for me. when people would slam their doors in her and my mom's face, when my family would come and try to mediate & talk to their parents. a lot of them showed no type of compassion, where I grew up was really insensitive, especially to me. it wasn't their child so they just didn't care the teasing and the bullying continued. nowhere to run. it just wasn't meant for me. it was meant for me to live not die I guess. at the age of 10 I attended a Japanese restaurant for the very 1st time in downtown Boston with my friend patan. it happened to be her 11th birthday and I had never seen Japanese food cooked and prepared in front of me inside the actual restaurant before. we ate with the chopsticks and all! it was fun and enlightening to me, and I enjoyed myself. it's such a long journey to me and it looks like there's no end to it anytime soon. I can thank the lord for that, some saw me as thinking that I am different & inferior to them I guess because of the alopecia but I am happy for all that have alopecia & those who don't equally. if I could have one wish I would hope one day that it gets better for the people with alopecia in this world. some type of breakthrough cure for this hair disease is what I would like to see. I would never know how it feels to go to the salon with a friend or family member and use the dryer, or get a wash like everyone else. more, people would randomly ask me "is that your hair?" and I would say "yes, I payed for it" I would say to myself in my mind "there is a whole different world out there". the alopecia community is a special place to me, I am just constantly thinking of more ways to educate & add knowledge on & make it better from when they first starting collecting data on this disorder in 1912 up until now. much hasn't changed as people have gotten wiser throughout time. as we know, it is a lifetime sickness but not life threating. that's actually where we fight half of the battle in this journey, as we walk through it together. I don't want you to be afraid, we can go through it all together. it feels like a different me, to feel what they are feeling out there at the same time they are. you may be scared and ashamed but you shouldn't be. be strong and smart, that is what counts. I can remember the day when one of the people that always wanted to be trouble to me met one of my family members. we saw her when she got off the bus the fight began as soon as her feet touched the sidewalk. that was one day I didn't have to worry about them, some of them would leave me alone after that incident but I was still scared out of my mind. but what could I do? I was a freightened little girl who avoided going where the bullies were. as long as they could not see me, then, they would not tease me anymore. I could never think right in them days my nerves were bad, and I was a scared little girl. trying to make friends but I always had the man upstairs to talk to when no one else would listen and understand me, he understood me. as I went to summer camp at the good will camp in new hampshire. we were in the woods, living in cabins. I didn't really like it, although it was only for 2 weeks. I was so scared, what about my hair? that's what I said to myself, here we go. time to take a shower and the girls standing around me trying to see what's under my shower cap. nosey skeezers! that was the worse. but you knew back in them days what types of different kinds of hairstyles were popular in the hood at the time. and then they'd go talking about me when we went to day camp at saint Patrick's. once, we went on a field trip to Houghton's pond in Milton, Massachusetts not knowing what I know today, as far as there being a whirlpool inside the pond. everyone was getting ready to swim and I went too deep into the water and almost drowned. I can remember looking up into the sky as the water sank into my mouth & my nose. I had gone too far out into the pond. one of the older guys came out to help me but the friend I thought had my back really didn't. not sure if my wig under the cap was a mess. my wig had a nasty look & when I got home my grandma said "what happened to your hair?" I said "I almost drowned in Houghton's pond, one of the older guys saved my life!" he was my hero that day to me but I thank the lord! I remember going down into the water and feeling like I was not coming back up but he saved my life that day he knows who he is. next day, I went to my 1st big modeling contest with a girl that I knew from around the area. it occurred at the Bradford hotel, it was a special place to me. coming from the projects, that was a good start for us. those were my dreams in them days the whole time it was like lights, camera, action we were the starlight's of the town that night. it was nearing the end of the competition & my friend was announced the winner. she had such a beautiful gown on and she was beautiful too. so it all fit together. I was happy for her saying to myself what's next for me? all I knew was that one day my grandma said to my mom "them girls are going to stop bullying her, she's going to karate school". so that was where I went next saying "this may help me". I finished karate school later that season. I still felt like I really didn't learn much though, just thinking they kept me there because I was out of harm's way doing something all of the time . . . patan & my other friend's buildings being so close together next to mine that we could see into each other's room, I vividly remember looking outside my window into one of my friend's window all the time. she would call me on the phone when this specific guy was there with her.

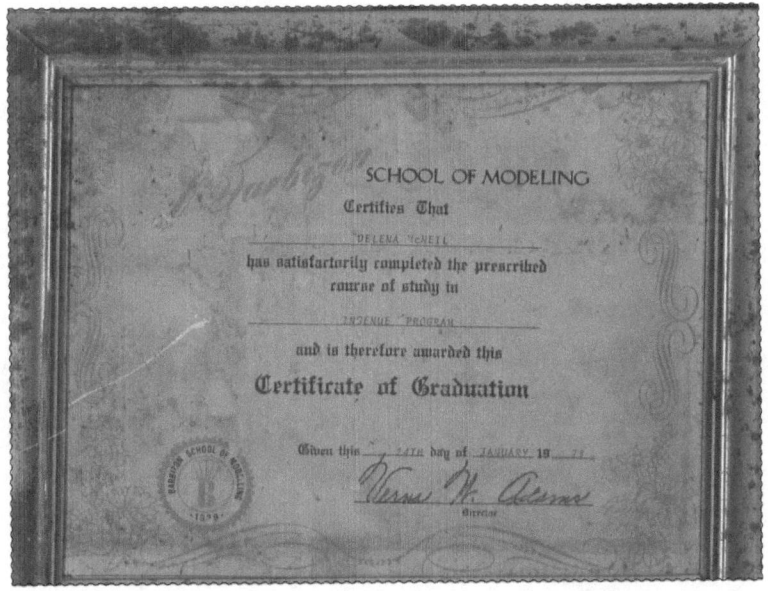

It happened to be one of the members of the new edition rib group. they were in the room and that was why I would only see shadows. anyway, my grandma sent me to barbizon modeling school, one of the best in the world. I did that and I finshed, but I didn't continue in the modeling field due to the fact that they wanted everything of mine to be really mine, including my hair. I just still couldn't find myself, still thinking & growing up feeling depressed and in hell having nightmares all the time. all my life I always wanted to know why I had to be different? will my kids be like this or what? I personally know now that most African American 's hair specifically is highly texturized & dry. these are 2 of the main things that make our hair more vunrable to breakage & also hair damage. I knew a lot of black girls when I was younger

& even now who would perm their hair, not knowing that these harsh chemicals cause permanent hair loss. there's also something called "androgenic alopecia" which mostly affects women who are entering the menopause stages. I really did not know if my baby would have the same hair problem I have being born. around the time I turned 15, my mother took us to canobie lake and we would have cookouts with our family there. I remember once my uncle slick got rained on with bird fecees on his shirt and all the kids were laughing. later on that year around holiday season we would all gather together for thanksgiving at grandma's house. everyone would bring food, although she would cook enough to feed everyone that showed up and then some. and on Christmas my grandmother had a white Christmas tree with a big black angel on the top of the tree to top the cultural empowerment that she stood for. my grandmother working the night shift and the determination she had being a single parent wasn't overlooked by me. she worked extra hard to provide for all of us and intend on carrying on tradition. I then started to become more acknowledged about being a girl, & becoming a young lady. hanging out with my cousin Sheila, we'd go and pick up cosmetics together. she would always insist on trying out new facial creams and she was always very adventurous. she was one of the first people to go into a wig store with me besides my mom and grandma. my mother would say that I was starting to "smell myself". there were a lot of crazy things going on in orchard park at this time, specifically, I still went through bullying with the other students though. we were all on the bus ride home & we went underneath a tunnel on the freeway. someone reached over from the seat behind me and snatched my wig off. I was embarrassed, I started crying and I didn't want to ride the bus anymore. so there were parent/teacher conferences after this incident which led to wild goose trails, no one would ever fess up to the wrongdoing done to me. during the 1980's my uncles, who were then collectively known as the "Cadillac boys" were among the elite of what was going on in the streets. one day there was a shootout in my mom's house. it was between my uncles and a few of their friends. all I remember was my mother holding me through it all. the Boston police came because there was a man lying dead in a pool of blood shot 3 times in my aunt's kitchen. it all started because one of the friends had a bit too much to drink, & they were all at my uncle's girlfriend's place. there was an argument over my uncle not wanting my mom to date his friend, and the guy made the biggest mistake of punching 1 of the Cadillac boys in the face & paid the ultimate price. 2 of my uncles were shot in the shootout as well, although they were not killed. one of them still has the bullet from that day inside of his back till this very day, and he walks & talks normal. doctors said that it would be to fatal to remove, being so close to his spine and all. that was just one story of many though. my grandmother was originally from Charleston, north Carolina. she was a mother of 6 children, 5 boys & 1 girl, my mother. I would periodically take trips with my 5 cousins and spend weeks down south in north Carolina from time to time. grandma would get on the train with us from Boston to Charleston, and even on the trains I would notice that people would stare at me and whisper. "why does she have a wig on at that age?" when I was down south that was the only place I didn't get picked on, that's why I used to like it down there. but it was much more country and slower paced than my usual Roxbury, Massachusetts city surroundings. one thing about my grandma was that she always made sure we were in church on Sundays, whether it was down south or in Boston. she was a very generous person, "blessed" to say the least. we grew up as Baptist Christians in our family as our religion. it was the 4th of July. we were all at my auntie cash's house & this was one of the 1st times I realized I was becoming a woman. I loved the way auntie cash's house was, she always had all the new video games, all the latest gadgets & she was always the nicest person's house to be at. we were playing tag, a game that you have to be physical in and I wasn't feeling too well. I needed to go to the restroom & I had a nausea like feeling in my cervical area, when I made it inside the stall I realized that I was bleeding. I didn't know it but this was the beginning of my womanhood. and then the conversations started. my grandmother insisted that I stayed away from boys. I would hear her & my mom talking to each other about me saying "you better watch her, she can get pregnant now running around with them lil' boys". at the beginning of august of that year, my sister & I went to stay with our cousins Melinda & shaker in Albany, new York. their mother worked during the day so we were left with the house to ourselves more often than not. their younger brother, my cousin romey was always incarcerated. he was a good young brother who was targeted by the local police department they always said. they would have friends over & loud hip hop music playing. I remember vividly hearing the sounds of Tina Marie, & the song "Roxanne, Roxanne" was one that I heard for the 1st time while I was there. they were into the Muslim religion at that time, and not eating pork. they were praying as Muslims 3 times a day, and this was a new experience to me. growing up believing in god and Jesus, it blew my mind to see my cousins so devoted to this. they would even tease me kind heartedly saying "you got that pig on your lips" referring to the fat inside the oil from the lipstick. that end of the summer trip with my sis to new York was much needed, only because I knew there would be much teasing & taunting to look forward to my freshman year at Charlestown high. as I entered high school I still had a difficult time learning. when it was time to switch classes people would whisper & point at me. freshman year was very rough, I felt like teachers were just giving me passing grades out of sympathy. sometimes I wished I could just go to the principal's office & get certain students' parents' contact info but we were in high school now & I didn't want to look too timid. softmore year breezed passed, I decided to enroll in a new advanced education honor class system. it meant taking college course subjects as my major studies that year. in my junior year I enrolled in a "work study" program, where I would go to school half the day & the other half I'd work a part time job at a restaurant & retail store. I went to the senior prom at Brighton high school with my uncle's girlfriend's brother. I really didn't want to go but she insisted, she bought me a dress, nails, perfume and all just to go. it was nice there, we danced and ate carved roast beef & salad for dinner. after the prom he asked me "do you think I can see you again?" and I replied "I don't know, I don't think so. but you're a nice guy & I had a good time". at this point I was starting to notice that guys were starting to look at me more like a real woman instead of just "girl Mrs. besley". at this time I was starting to take pride in my appearance more. girls would notice me doing little upgrades on my appearance whether the new pair of sunglasses, new clothes, or even a new wig, they would be jealous. I wouldn't usually hang out in orchard park much anymore. my friends & I would go on our adventures to blue hill ave, sneaking out to smoke cigarettes & drink small nip bottles of liquor. we would get packs of free cigarettes because companies would just hand them out at the parks in our part of the city, even to children under 18. I believe that's how a lot of people in the black community became so dependent on certain cigarette brands. the trains that would ride over Roxbury would have massive grafitti on them when they went by. I remember a lot of people got robbed by orchard park residents until they took the train service away from Roxbury altogether. once, I remember some guys stealing a whole rack of mink coats from a store and running into the projects with the coats still on the rack. as soon as they were spotted by us coming into the projects they dissappeared, and then the feds came in knocking on doors, including ours. "we're doing an investigation on the theft of the mink coats that were taken from goldie's fur coat store in the south end" I remember the captain saying. after that night the assailants were never caught or prosecuted for the coats. there were nice days sometimes in the projects too though sometimes. I was there on the day one of michael bivins' relatives graduated high school. it was a late model pearl white rolls royce driven by a spiffy dressed chauffeur. he opened the door and people started taking pictures of it as she got in. she was wearing the same creamish-pearl colored gown that the vehicle was painted. I can just still see the orange leather interior and remember the smoke from the white wall tires driving out of the projects, as she waved at us and continued on her way. after awhile new edition became very successful, and sold tens of millions of records worldwide. they would sit on my grandmother's stoop long before they got their 1st record deal and practice singing. it would upset her because she worked the night shift 11-7 as a nurse's assistant in the trauma unit at Boston city hospital. it was the mid 80's and everyone was getting ready to graduate high school or going to college. meanwhile, I was pregnant. I was getting ready to have a child with a man who wasn't bothered by my alopecia or what people said about me, he saw the beauty in me that was always there. then my son was born and I was very ecstatic to know that he was born without the alopecia disease. I remember being thankful to the lord for that, I always wondered throughout the pregnancy how it would turn out and it turned out for the better, god was definitely on my side! I was at home for awhile nurturing my newborn. trying to find my place in the world under a new title, mother. as I did, I would fill out applications for various retail store & fast food businesses until one hired me. I had dropped out of high school after finding out I would have to support a baby. I always thrived off of independence. I utilized the transitional assistance program for awhile, and after living house to house I ended up pregnant again. this was when I moved to a small town in the southern part of Massachusetts called fall river. the 90's had moved in, my oldest son was just starting headstart and my 2nd child had just been born, I was just so overwhelmed with joy for him, he was born with so much hair! we began seeing my sons' father's relatives a lot more often than I saw mine. I would only see my relatives around the holidays like Christmas, and that began to be a real problem to me. I noticed more after the 2nd child, another beautiful healthy baby boy, that the father became somewhat more controlling. in clubs or even at train stations, at stores he would get violent with men who would try to say things to me or even men who just looked at me. as I felt like the relationship was going downhill, I began to stay at my mother's and grandmother's house. he would come by my mother's and they would tell him to not be so violent. as time went by my relationship with Mr. man vanished, and I began a new life. I sat and said to myself "it's time to close this chapter and start a new one". I called a cab company one Friday morning after packing all of what the children & I needed. our clothes, bottles of milk, animal crackers, their toys and gameboys. I was waiting all day at the DTA office patiently because I new it was crowded, and back then we didn't have cell phones. told the transitional assistance worker that "I have 2 kids & I can only stay at my mother's for a week & we need somewhere to go" she said "well, its 4:30 in the afternoon and we can't find a placement for you at this time" that's when I said "well we're all packed up, I just did the laundry, bottles are filled with milk . . . I guess we'll just go with you Mrs. davis!". she replied "oh wait! hold on Mrs. smith. we'll figure something out . . . just sit down . . . let me make a few calls. I waited another 15-20 minutes while she franticly dialed numbers & pressed the hang up button to dial more. before I knew it, they placed me in a battered women's shelter, in the south end section of Boston. we were there for about 6 months. then we went to the town line inn in saugus, mass. we were there about 6 months as well. after our stint in the various shelters, a few apartment management companies started to take me for occupancy interviews. eventually I found something on ruthven street in

Roxbury. my younger brother angel would come over and babysit for me when I needed him to. just to give me a break from the boys every now and then, for a small fee. I didn't mind though because I knew the kids would be in good hands and I knew he was in prep school and he needed money for college. he graduated from thayer academy high school and played on the basketball team for the school as well. he furthered his education, going to college to get a bachelor's in psycology. seeing that made me very proud as a big sister, and reassured me that dreams do come true, even for project kids like us. it was a lot of drug dealing, violent crimes, gang activity, killings, etc. there but it was our very own apartment after all we had gone through together. we struggled in the beginning & I got a lot of the 1st few pieces of furniture from second hand non profit organizations that were steppingstones along the way. soon I landed a gig for a temp agency working at the prudential building & I came across a $4,000 cash settlement from a car accident to purchase a new vehicle and stablize things more for me and my children. as my life became more interesting, I began meeting my new neighbors and peers in the neighborhood. I would hang out with girlfriends at local nightclubs like slades, & the barritz on the weekends. we would usually hit the after hours burger shops like the whopper spot in the wee hours of the morning. then it was time to go home, to eat a bit more and take care of the children after getting much needed rest. as I fall asleep, I fell off into a reminiscent dream of what my 16th birthday was like. my mom, grandmom, & auntie cash threw me a "sweet 16 party" in the projects. we stayed on the 3rd floor and my grandmother lived on the 1st floor in the adjacent building that connected to ours. at some point during the night there were 2 people who got robbed on the 1st floor at gunpoint in my mom's building while my party was going on, that ended the party. word was that they were robbed because they were sticking people up around the way & they happened to be wearing new bomber coats, which were very popular leather coats at the time. my auntie cash and uncle blue decided to take us to the wax museum one day in downtown Boston. as we entered the museum, I was scared out of my mind after seeing the 1st 3 wax figures, as they hang horrificly from the ceiling. I stayed outside of the building looking at the clock on the church across the street until my cousin maxwell, joy, & my lil' sis came out of the museum. after we went to the museum we would often go to a downtown family owned restaurant my cousin maxwell liked to eat at. a few days later there was another shootout around my mom's building. they must've been on the roof or in another apartment when it happened, but someone was shooting and a bullet went inside my mother's house through the wall. it went from the living room wall to the wall in the kitchen. after this, something happened that changed the way I looked at the projects. I heard silence & you could hear a pin drop, this was unheard of in my neighborhood. I didn't know how to handle the silence so I got up & went to the window to see what had happened. there were people standing around in a very circular crowd, not to overshadow the 4 people in the middle of the circle. there was a short man, very well dressed & decked in gold. 3 gold chains, a gold rolex, & a handful of rings. his pockets were all bulging with knots of cash, and I can hear people say "that's him . . . that's him . . . that's allah". he had snapped his fingers and that had been the reason for the silence, I never saw anyone have so much control of entire violent project like that before. there were 2 guys holding a man up bleeding from his nose and mouth. I guess the man owed some money to them & allah said "beat his ass" and they followed his orders. I had no idea at this time that I was watching how the new biggest heroin empire head was running things. they were called "the apple boys" because they originally came from the big apple I assume. this is when I noticed that orchard park was changing for the worse. even though allah ruled with an iron fist, they did do some good things for the younger kids around the project. I remember on labor day the apple boys rented yellow school buses and took 90% of the children in the projects on a trip to six flags great adventure in jackson, new jersey. even a few of my little cousins, who were in their teens at the time had gone with them on that trip. my mother and grandmother were asking me if I knew where they were and I had no idea because I knew nothing about what was going on. all I remember was them coming back later on that day with hats and big stuffed animals and accessories you knew they had got them at the theme park. they were still so hyped up and eager to tell us about the rides they had got on and which ones were the scariest. I was happy to see that they were alright & they had a good time, but I thought it must've been pretty cool for them to have the chance to see another environment. even if it was just for a day, they got a chance to look at something other than orchard park which was important to me. six months later, there was a huge drug sweep in orchard park, which was televised on national television, & then years later developed into a full length box office motion picture release. this was the time I met another man that thought outside the box, with a different background and upbringing than me. he was from a household that actually lived in a house, his name was Mr. smooth. his family lived there and his mom & dad were still together. he even worked a legitimate job. coming from my upbringing it was a new experience for me. since I was living at 128 ruthven street my friend patat stayed with us for a few weeks to help warm up the house and make it more home like and comfortable, which was located right off of humboldt ave. it was a very drug infested neighborhood. soon after, my youngest sister cocoa came to stay with me from Albany. she was staying with my father and we discussed me being in her life more as a big sister. we figured it would be good for her, being that she was getting older into her teens being 16 in the mid 90's, it was getting very dangerous in Albany at that time and she was at risk. it was nice for me to be able to help my dad out and take care of her for him. my sister, being mulatto, there was a lot of envy towards her from the other full blooded African American tennage females when she came to live with me in the neighborhood that I lived in being from out of town to begin with, and then based on her lighter skin & naturally wavy straight hair, we have the same dad but her mother was caucasion. one day as baby sis was sitting on the stoop outside she met a new friend named tammy, who she later found out lived right next door to us and I was very close to tammy's mother. the 2 of them got to be very close friends over time, going to the movies together, shopping, and hanging out together at the house. after about 5 years of going through those things and learning from me more how to survive as an adult, baby sis went and moved to troy, new York to live, and also pursued school and a career in medical assisting. she also moved back to be closer to our father and take care of him more wich made me proud, since Albany was less than an hour away. after baby sis left, tammy continued school and soon graduated high school. after getting a degree in the medical field, she became a 1st time homeowner as well as a mother herself. I learned to get along though and my new boyfriend mr smooth began to come around more often. he would help with groceries, & at the time I had just got my new car so he helped me pick new tires and he kept it washed and looking clean because it was a white car after all. we had our fair share of disagreements, but overall we found a common ground to build foundation upon. people would continuosly try to persuade him to leave me because of my hair disease, he would laugh it off and tell me it was only because they wanted a chance to date me. after a couple of years went by and the relationship started evolving, the family grew once again and I had my 3rd child in November of 1993, who also like my 2nd was born with a head full of hair. again, I thanked the lord having another healthy baby with 5 fingers and 5 toes. after I had my 1st child with Mr. smooth and he became more familiar with my family, I found out that he had a child from a previous relationship and he started to bring his son around more to play with mine.

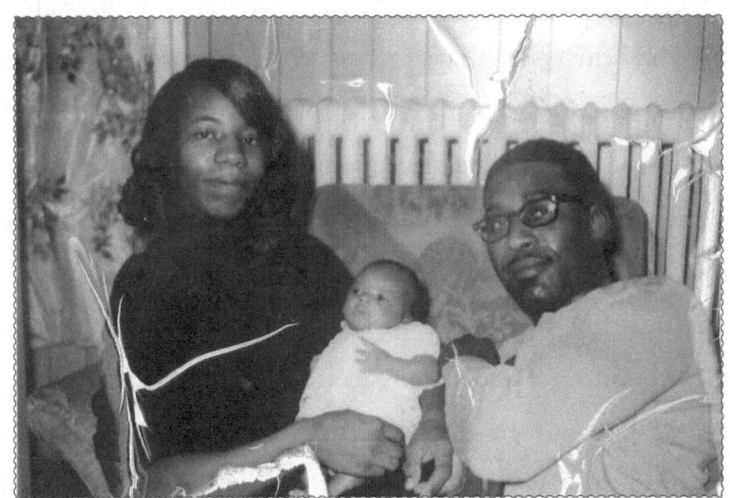

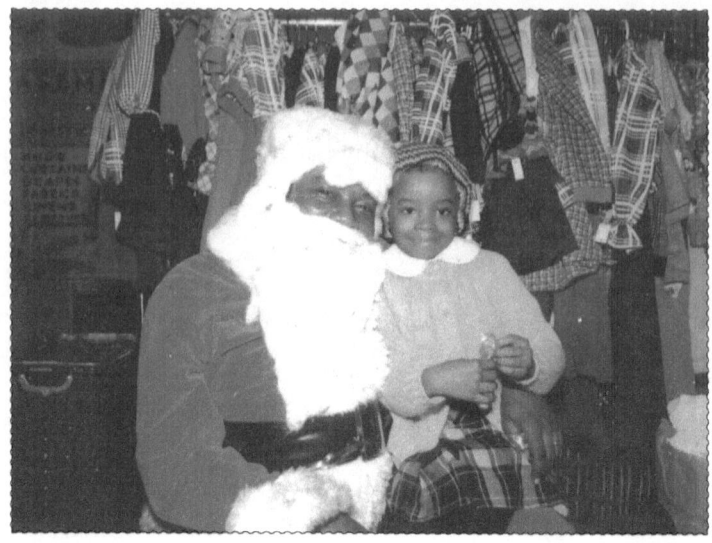

We would start to spend holidays together and go to his parents' house for dinners on thanksgiving & Christmas, there would always be gifts for my children. his parents did for mr smooth's son from the previous relationship & mine just the same. going into the new year my apartment management notified me of new renovation plans for the building, as well as relocation plans for the tenants, like myself. we then moved to the codman square neighborhood on Melbourne street. we were there for about 2 years, we had our good & bad days there. looking back, on Melbourne street was the last time I can recall physically seeing & speaking to my younger cousin Carlton and it was my 1st time finding out that he had just become a new father and he was going to bring his newborn son by to see me, he never made it back. he was the oldest and there was his younger brother, my other cousin

Maurice. I didn't know all of the details until later but Carlton was on the run at the time for violating the rice drug laws. they accused him of being a kingpin in dealing heroin. he was caught with a kilogram of it and was given a life sentence with no possiblity of parole. after losing his big brother Carlton my younger cousin Maurice ended up following in his big brother's foot steps. in & out of prison throughout his early 20's, he became well known for drug dealing & robberies. my oldest son was in his teens at this time & was becoming negatively active in the neighborhood, getting into fights with the new neighbors' children. we eventually moved back to the Roxbury section of Boston into a townhouse on seaver street in the year 2000. being back on our side of town and on seaver street specifically, we were able to go on our balcony and see all of the always crowded city's annual festivals, for the Caribbean, Puerto Rican, & Dominican heritages in the city, when they didn't turn into fights & shootouts. by this time my 2nd son started to get to that age where he was approaching his early teen years. so now there were 3 teenagers in the house, let alone the neighborhood we lived in. the boys kept me going, as smooth jr. was getting ready to graduate high school I figured we'd go to pick out a suit together for his senior prom. after that, he got a rent-a-car for the occasion to go along with his nice girl he was taking. after prom he focused on a career in the new digital music industry, studying at local community colleges, although he left after a few semesters. he went on to do deejaying work with various artists and execs at venues across the country and then out of nowhere I got pregnant. in the summer of 2001 Mr. smooth & I decided that we were going to take our family of 7, including all of the children on an all expense paid, poolside hotel stay, family trip. we went to Florida, Kissimmee is where Disney world was. we stayed at the holiday express, which had a special set up for children. it was equipped with video games & pizza. we were there for a week, we took the family to Disney world while we were in town. we went to just about every division that the world famous amusement park had to offer. then Mr. smooth surprised us all with a surprise dinner at red lobster. I can just still see the giant alien cups that stood at least 2 feet tall that the kids were drinking out of, each child had one. we both knew that since our boys were getting older the Florida trip would be 1 of the last times the family would all be together in one place at one time. we were right, the older boys began working part time jobs which became full time very soon after. we then decided that it was time for the parents to go on a trip. my sister in law watched the kids & we went to Bermuda for 6 nights and 7 days. it was beautiful, the scenery took my breath away. we found out that they drove with the steering wheel on the other side of the car. my sister & her husband attended as well with Mr. smooth and I. we were all on a cruise ship & we were playing bingo and gambling on most nights. it was really nice, they had a nice nightclub we went to drinking and dancing through the night. we drove the 4 wheelers and had a good time going through the various attractions the island of Bermuda had to offer. for the last 2 nights we went to the casino and won on the slot machines. I won money on the machines when we first arrived in Bermuda & my sis won some on our trip back home to the united states. I was blessed again in august of 2001 with a healthy baby boy who was born with a head full of hair, I named him Ricky. Ricky turned out to be a fast learner from the start, taking to sports by age 3. playing in leagues by age 5 & receiving awards at that age in football & baseball. shortly after my 4th son was born we went to Albany, new York so that my great grandmother on my father's side could see the new baby as well as a preview of the next generation. my sons were infatuated with the idea that people can live that long and make it to that age, she was 99 at the time. I wanted to show them also where their mother was born. on the trip I just reminisced on fun times with great grandma at her house. my 3rd boy started to get older as well. not only that, he paid very good attention to what was being done around him. I always tried to keep my children active in whatever community activity programs or overnight camps that were fun and out of the area. summer basketball leagues, the aquarium, the movies, the circus, and it seemed like there was always a birthday party going on twice per month. who knows who was eating cake out of all the out of household attendees. but we didn't care about the money, we just wanted to see our children happy and show them other things. live a better life, but I also wanted them to see that there was more to life than what they saw outside everyday. the oldest was into sports like basketball & education in his teens mostly, although he did drop out of school eventually without my best wishes of course. then one of my son's friends ended up getting pistol whipped in front of the building and management decided it would be a good idea for them to terminate our agreement, after 15 years of being a tenant for them. we moved in about a week, we relocated to Brockton, mass. our new location had its festivities as well to enjoy, we would see the fireworks being lit on the 4th of July. I liked the new hardwood floor and figured that the apartment had potential. we spent 1 Christmas there but we all enjoyed our 1st trip to the Brockton fair that year. we would have cookouts in the backyard when the weather was nice. what we didn't realize was that there were so many health code violations with the house where we were living & we would soon have to vacate the premises due to negligence of the landlord. the 2 youngest boys and myself were put into a transitional housing program through ymca. after 6 months I moved to another landlord's property. it was around may 2008 and it was just about time for me to run and check the mail. I was going downstairs and my neighbors had family over and there were kids running around in the front hall. when I went outside to check the box I had noticed one of the children was still in the car(mini van) and would not get out. when I was looking into the car to see her I saw a beautiful little girl with a scarf on her head and she wasn't saying anything, she was just looking outside the window. I said "hello pretty mama" and went back upstairs but it did stay on my mind. the whole night I said to myself I'd ask my neighbor about the little girl the next time I see her. when I saw her and asked her about it she told me that the girl did in fact have alopecia, and that's what I was saying to myself the whole night I knew it. after seeing this problem in kids it hurt me inside even more and made me want to try to do something that would benefit people around the world, educating them on the disease. it reminded me that I don't deal with this alone and there are plenty of beautiful babies like that affected by this. all the training that I received from the adult education center (the ambro academy) I felt that I failed at, as well as cali for nail academy I felt I that I failed. also, when I worked for anodyne corportion as a temp employee I felt that it failed to give me what I feel I deserved. I felt that I could never find myself until I started writing. that was when I found myself, and I thank the lord for my blessing. medical coding and billing failed. maybe the lord had other plans and this is it I hope. when I went to the doctor for a routine check up, he startled me saying that he was setting me up for an mri. I went for my back and my neck. as I got into the machine it started to pull me in. it pulled my hair/wig and once again even in my adulthood I felt embarrassed like when I was a kid.

After dealing with MRI results now I find out that my landlord happened to misinform the inspectors that my family occupied the top floor apartment as well as the one I was in, which wasn't a true statement for him to tell the inspectors. The top floor apartment was where an entirely different family of another nationality resided. The landlord was subsequently arrested and prosecuted. We decided it would be best for me to find a better landlord to deal with, and in turn, we moved into a bat cave like undisclosed location in Brockton, which wasn't as worse as the previous landlords' properties. Once we got things settled I landed a job, and then another night shift job. Things were going good for a while then I was in a serious car accident. This made it so I couldn't work both jobs anymore and doctors told me "no more strenuous work anymore". I started therapy with physical therapists 3-4 times a week for my injuries. One day the Brockton police came to my residence looking for my eldest son. He had broke a fraction of rules from a previous charge, this caused attention to my family from neighbors and the landlord as well. We had a meeting with the landlord in which representatives from the housing program attended. The topic of discussion was my children . . . my boys. I had a glimpse of returning to a transitional housing shelter if the meeting didn't go well, but thank the lord that it did. My son began getting into more mischief, getting caught up into incarceration for continuing the criminal lifestyle. With a child always away in jail, it hurts but I had time to focus and analyze life a bit more, personally. it was like the sight of my own life was starting to become clearer to me. as I would speak to him over the phone and send him cash for food & personal cosmetics when I was able to, these are the things that reminded me of my purpose as a mother in this world no matter what happens. also, that life still goes on after alopecia and there are always going to be other tougher obstacles put in front of us to go through. the important thing I believe is to look past the obstacles at our goals to work towards a good future. as long as you got the good lord on your side, it is impossible to go wrong. one of my all time dreams is to own my own salon for people with alopecia as well as design and create my own wig line. I would want the wigs to be unisex so that both men, women, & children could wear them.

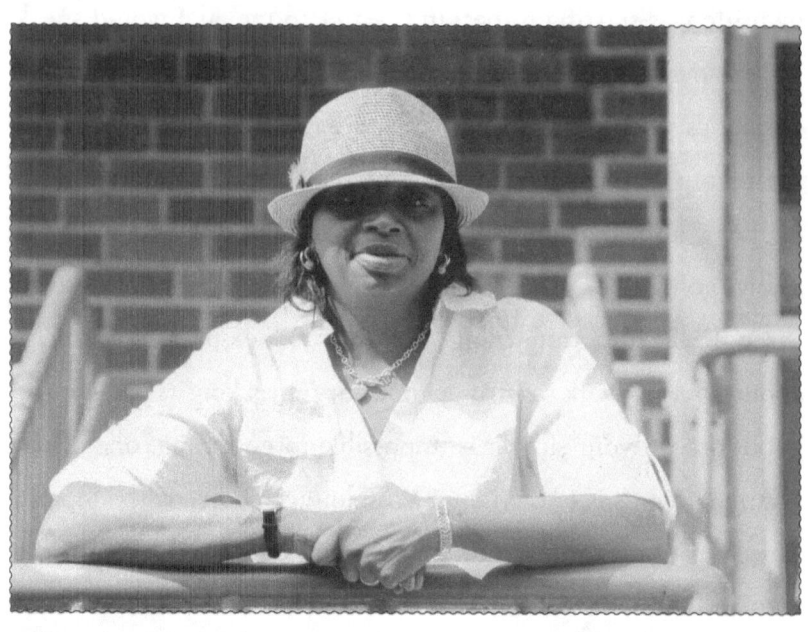

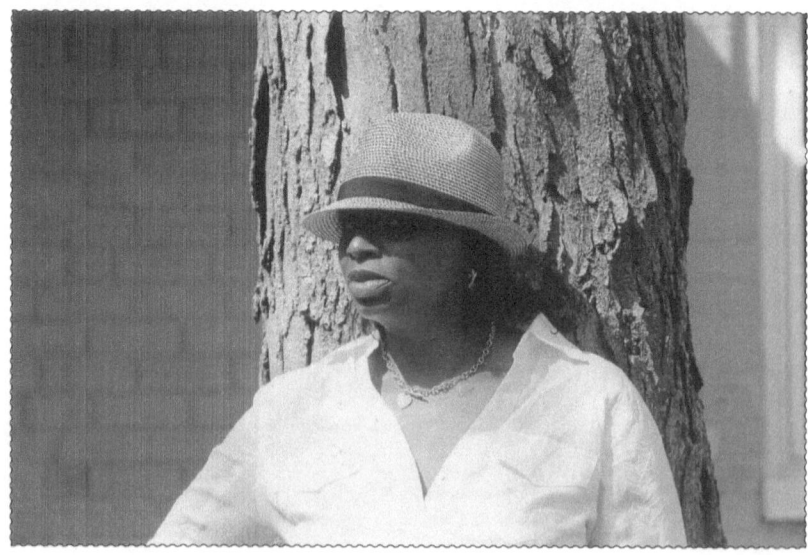

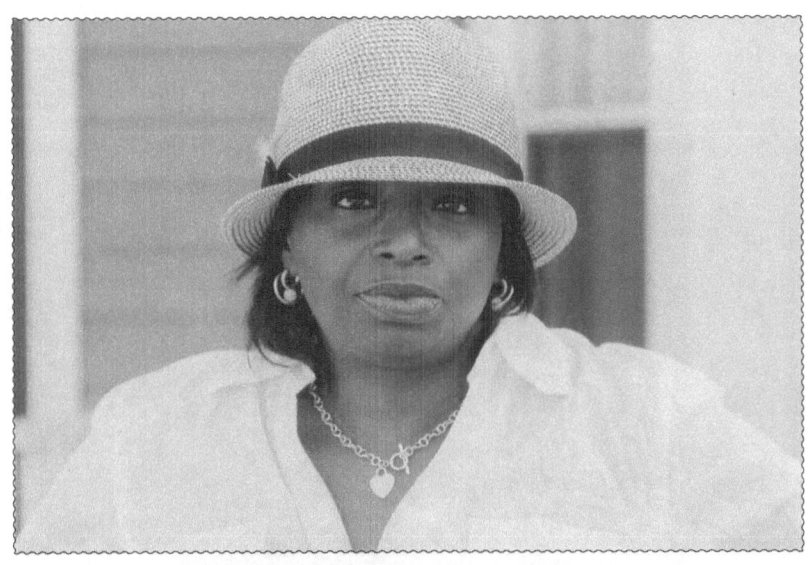

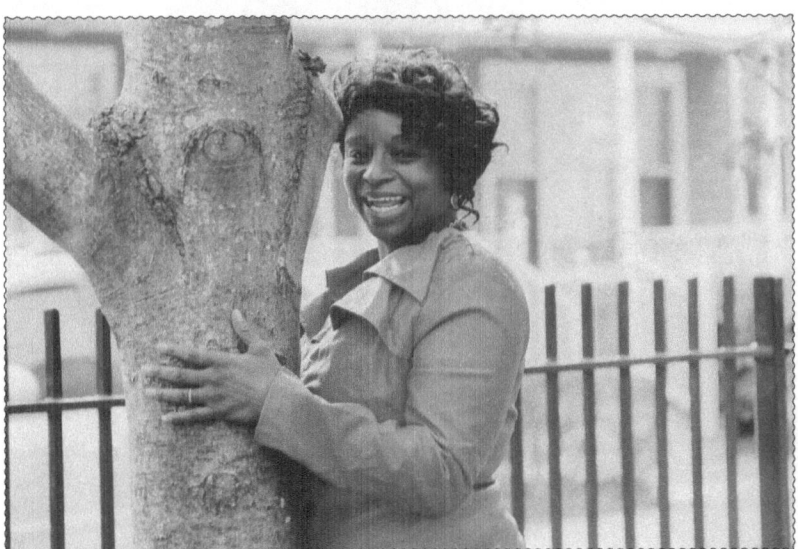

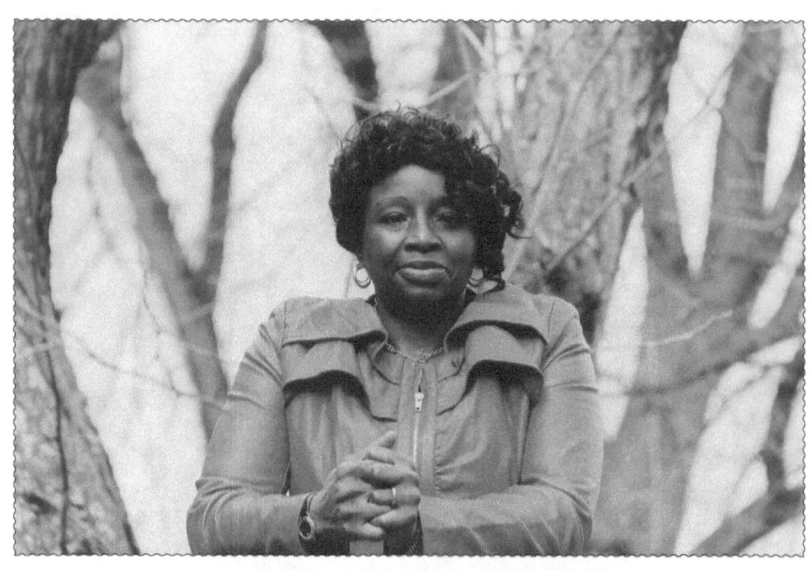

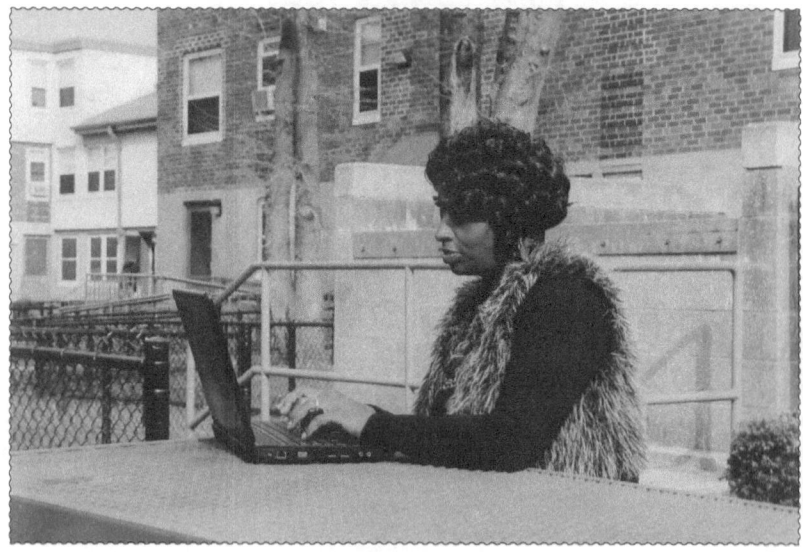